Deirdre Earls, MBA, RD, LD

Your Healing Diet

Austin

This book is written for Pop because I promised him that someday I'd write a book.

Thank you for sharing your time and please let me know how I can help you to experience the incredible healing power of food!

Deirdre Earls, MBA, RD, LD
www.YourHealingDiet.com
(512) 453-8784

To order additional copies, please contact us.
BookSurge
www.booksurge.com
1-866-308-6235
orders@booksurge.com

Table of Contents

Introduction   vii

Chapter One: Taking Control of Your Health   1

Chapter Two: The Big Experiment   5

Chapter Three: How Food Can Create and Reverse
                    Disease…Slowly   9

Chapter Four: Healing Principles – Diet, Positive
                    Outlook, Activity   15

Chapter Five: The Acid/Alkaline Balance & Why a
                    Healing Diet Works   21

Chapter Six: Healing Diet Basics   25

Chapter Seven: Grocery Shopping   37

Chapter Eight: In My Refrigerator   45

Chapter Nine: In Austin Restaurants   49

Chapter Ten: On a Trip   49

Chapter Eleven: What to Expect   57

Chapter Twelve: Easy, Recipe-free Meals and
Snacks   61

Introduction:

"It would be possible to describe everything scientifically, but it would make no sense; it would be without meaning, as if you described a Beethoven symphony as a variation of wave pressure." Albert Einstein

This guidebook is written to inspire you to experience the incredible healing power of food in the midst of very busy lifestyles. I invested hundreds of hours learning the shortcuts on how to research, shop, travel, cook and dine differently in order to experience natural healing with food. To save you time and speed the benefits to you, I have distilled reams of information into this user-friendly, conversational guide.

Personal desperation initiated this journey. For thirty years I struggled with severe psoriasis. Despite fifteen years as a Registered Dietitian and thirty years of appointments with physicians around the world, I hadn't heard how food could be my medicine.

In June 2002 my condition worsened and the skin on my hands no longer allowed me to pick up a glass of water or open a jar. Expensive, chemotherapeutic drugs with horrible side effects had been recommended. In desperation I searched online and was introduced to a dietary approach that enables the body to heal itself. It was easy to understand why the diet supports natural healing. With nothing to lose but a disease and unwanted weight, I committed myself to this way of eating for six months. By December 2002 my hands had cleared almost completely. I also lost twenty pounds and spent no money on prescription medications.

There are many healing diets including Macrobiotics, Raw Foods, Alkalizing, Anti-inflammatory, Cancer Prevention, Heart Disease Prevention and Anti-Aging. These diets are associated with healing dozens of degenerative and autoimmune diseases. Like all of them, my approach to natural healing emphasizes whole grains, vegetables, legumes, fruits, nuts and seeds. Professional and personal experience showed me that they are rarely practiced because it is difficult to sustain good eating habits in the midst of busy lifestyles.

Although I respect the potential value of strict adherence to a healing diet, this book is written for those who have limited time to practice it completely. This guidebook is a "fast food" version of sorts, meaning that the information is adapted to fit a busy lifestyle while still helping the body to achieve levels of natural healing. I have never been 100% compliant, and I occasionally eat foods that are strongly discouraged. But to my surprise, my less than perfect practice achieves remarkable healing. I wrote this book to help others experience the incredible healing power of food in a way that doesn't require seismic shifts in every dimension of life.

This book is written as a brief guide. It is not a medical study. Views presented herein on the genesis of disease, how food can prevent and reverse disease, and the diet suggestions themselves are merely my interpretations of research and how natural healing happened for me. This book references a healing diet that's promoted by a top ranked American medical school but I make no claim this information is scientifically proven nor that this is a guaranteed cure. My intent is simply to illustrate how a quality diet can fit into a busy lifestyle, enhance quality of life and reduce healthcare expense while suffering no negative side effects. The choice is yours to decide if you will give food a chance to be your medicine.

Chapter 1
Taking Control of Your Health

"Liberty means responsibility. That is why most men dread it." George Bernard Shaw

With all the anxieties of any newly minted adolescent, I was thirteen and walking into my first day at Central Junior High School. One thing made me particularly self-conscious that day. Sometime over the preceding summer, severe psoriasis had erupted all over my body. Walking into a new school with hundreds of new faces, I knew I couldn't hide this reality. Quiet support from family and friends helped me to accept this problem and insist that it not rule my life.

Twenty-five years with psoriasis passed. Those years included two months in the hospital and thousands of dollars in drugs and doctors around the world. Some treatments would clear my skin for a couple of months, but quick relapses yielded a worsened condition. Powerful, expensive drugs emerged offering better results and terrible side effects.

During this time, I graduated with honors in Scientific Nutrition from Texas A&M University. After completing a dietetic internship at The Indiana University Medical Center, I practiced as a Registered Dietitian for almost fifteen years. Throughout this twenty year phase of my career, I heard nothing of what diet could do for my skin.

The turning point came in June of 2002. All of a sudden I couldn't unscrew jars or pick up a glass of water. Knuckles started to look arthritic and simply turning a steering wheel opened cracks in my hands. I was desperate and knew that a trip to the doctor would yield a prescription for methotrexate, a chemotherapy used to treat breast cancer. Like other prescription medication options for psoriasis, it offers brief relief, long-term side effects, and costly medical bills.

Anxious to be free of strong prescription medications, I went online and started searching for anything related to psoriasis. To my surprise, "diet" started appearing. Several sources taught me that psoriasis happens when one eats foods to which they have an allergy or sensitivity. Perhaps in conjunction with an acid-forming diet and proliferation of damaging intestinal microbes, the allergic response renders a "leaky gut". Subsequent toxic seepage leads to a series of autoimmune responses, the consequences of which can be psoriasis or many other degenerative diseases like arthritis, heart disease, diabetes, and cancer.

With nothing to lose, I committed myself to natural healing with food. At first I was amazed at how much better I felt. Then I was struck at how quickly friends told me that my entire persona was changing. I embarked upon hundreds of hours in research and cooking classes that taught me how to use food to heal. The more I practiced a healing diet, the faster my skin healed. Sometimes the new demands and requisite patience were overwhelming, but encouragements to persevere kept me focused.

Symptoms sometimes worsen before they improve when one pursues natural healing. This happened to me and it took five months before my symptoms began to visibly improve. After six months, my hands and allergies had healed almost completely. Additionally, I had lost twenty pounds of unwanted weight and spent no money on prescription medications or physician appointments.

I have enormous gratitude for finding a solution that relieved my skin with no negative side effects, slashed my food and medical costs, helped me lose over twenty pounds, and set me free from dependency on doctors and drugs. I was inextricably drawn to share this diet and my knowledge in diet education to help others achieve the same benefits.

Personal experience and years of nutrition education taught me that even in desperate situations, dietary habits can be very difficult to change. My mission is to help you take control of your health via a diet that promotes natural healing and fits your busy lifestyle, thereby enhancing your compliance and probability for long-term success.

Chapter 2
The Big Experiment

"Take the first step in faith. You don't have
to see the whole staircase, just take the first
step." Martin Luther King, Jr.

After committing to a six month experiment to
see how diet might affect my psoriasis, I embarked
upon hundreds of research hours. The online information ranged from international medical sites to home
remedies to books. Across multitudes of sources, I
looked for common threads of success. I repeatedly
found the importance of avoiding animal products
(beef, pork, chicken and dairy), refined sugars, refined
flours, processed foods, alcohol, fatty foods, hydrogenated fats and overly spicy foods. There also seemed
to be a frequent connection between gluten intolerance and autoimmune problems like psoriasis. Being a
Texan with who favored meat, beer, and jalapenos as
dietary staples, it was anything but easy to part with
these foods. But the more I studied, the more I knew
that I had nothing to lose except a disease, unwanted weight and destructive habits. Additionally, it was
obvious that this diet would protect me from obesity,
heart disease, diabetes and cancer.

My first step towards practicing natural healing came after reading a book by Dr. John Pagano, a chiropractic physician. He teaches, "In essence, holistic healing is properly setting in motion the forces of nature within the individual that will help the body to heal itself." Dr. Pagano's recommendations include diet, enemas and colonics, spinal adjustments, various ointments and specific baths. Although I deeply appreciate the value of his work, I wasn't comfortable with some of his recommendations and subsequently focused solely on those which I knew to contribute no harm, namely the diet, an optimistic outlook and regular outdoor activity.

Within a week of diet change, I had a very deep and rare sense of knowing that I was doing the right thing. I could feel my whole body breathing a sigh of relief. Soon friends were commenting on my new "glow" and the positive change in my persona. I explained Dr. Pagano's diet and many likened it to other healing diets. Across much research I found that healing diets encourage a daily preponderance of vegetables and fruits. Most of them also appeared to take a severe stance towards compliance. Years of work as a hospital dietitian taught me the inefficacy of simply lecturing on radical diet change. Very few people adhere to strict diets for long periods of time. It is much more useful to educate on how to adapt a good diet to fit into one's personal lifestyle. This is especially true when attempting to achieve natural healing with food because this process is invariably slow and it requires great patience. For most of us, the process of healing with food is "two steps forward, one step back".

I continued researching all types of healing diets. Unlike Dr. Pagano's diet, many other healing diets exclude animal products, namely dairy, meats, fish and eggs. I decided to eliminate all animal products except fish as part of my experiment. To the extent that I restricted animal products from my diet, my skin and allergies cleared much more quickly. Whereas I didn't become and do not expect to become vegetarian nor vegan, I dramatically reduced my average intake of animal products. Because of the results, I've never turned back.

Importantly, I learned that a healing diet built upon fresh vegetables and fruit, whole grains, beans, lentils, nuts and seeds and occasional animal product is a way of eating that enhances health, prevents disease and promotes natural healing for everyone, not just for those with psoriasis.

Chapter 3
How Food can Create and Reverse Disease.... Slowly

"Success seems to be connected with action. Successful men keep moving. They make mistakes, but they don't quit." Conrad Hilton

In the first chapter I introduced a possible genesis of many diseases, namely that poor elimination and ingestion of certain foods and toxins can damage the lining of the intestines and create a leaky gut. In conjunction with an acid-forming diet and proliferation of damaging bacteria and parasites, toxins subsequently leak into the bloodstream and ultimately create overload on our filtering organs. The liver filters blood and the kidneys filter water. As the liver and kidneys are increasingly taxed with greater toxic volume, they start shuttling the extra toxins to other elimination organs like the skin and the lungs. Hence, our body alerts us to early stages of illness via discharge of these extra toxins at these areas. This is when we develop colds, sinus congestion, coughing, sneezing, excessive sweating and minor skin irritations. Unresolved seepage of pollutants from the intestines leads to further toxic build up in the body. Acute problems become chronic problems and generalized fatigue. If the cause of the problem is not corrected, the body's elimination methods are increasingly taxed and the body begins to accumulate more damaging levels of toxins at deeper levels. This yields more serious problems in other discharge areas of the body like ears, tonsils, uterus, sinuses, gums, lungs. Autoimmune disorders like arthritis, lupus, and shingles may develop at this stage of accumulation. Further toxic accumulation demands that the body store toxins in ever deeper areas, ultimately producing degenerative alterations in vital organs. Most major diseases including cancers, cardiovascular disease, and diabetes arise at this point. Some view these diseases as the body's natural means of isolating pollutants in tumors and organs instead of allowing toxins to systemically overwhelm the bloodstream, yielding more immediate death. This uncanny ability of our body not only "buys time" but also offers the opportunity to reflect on how our choices directly influence our condition and change according to the health we want.

Now that you understand this theory on the progression of disease, it's important to understand how food can reverse disease. First, by eliminating the foods which weaken the intestinal lining and feed bad microbes, you stop contributing to intestinal damage and provide necessary relief for healing of that tissue. As you stop the intestinal damage, you'll also halt the leaking of toxins and thereby give the body's filtration and immune systems a well deserved break. As your choices no longer contribute to an overtaxed immune system, you'll allow it to regain its ability to discharge toxins instead of storing them. And by including healing foods into your diet, you'll be providing the necessary nutrition and environment to build healthy tissue and blood. This renders natural healing throughout the body.

One of the wonderful things about natural healing is being able to view the sequential consequences of good decisions, and how good decisions perpetuate themselves with more positives. In other words, **to the extent that you demonstrate respect and gratitude for your body by making choices that nurture instead of damage it, you experience a long series of positive responses.** Almost immediately, you feel better and recognize the sense that you're doing the right thing.

However, despite this simple logic for natural healing, adopting this way of eating was anything but easy. It was the most difficult thing I have ever done because I was so attached to my old eating habits. The good news is that this new way of eating ultimately becomes its own habit, and you start to crave how quality food makes you feel. You recognize the difference in your energy, moods and vitality. To the extent that you are compliant, you will feel the difference. And this feeling will act as a strong motivator to keep you compliant long before you see symptom improvement.

It is important to mention that when one decides to address the cause of disease, one decides to go inward and heal more completely from the inside out versus simply addressing symptoms from the outside in. This inward discipline and natural healing requires time. The natural healing process is almost always slow. It requires patience, persistence and commitment. Natural healing is rarely an overnight phenomenon, so you shouldn't expect an immediate improvement in your symptoms. In general, the longer someone has experienced symptoms, the greater the extent of toxic accumulation and the longer it takes to discharge that accumulation from the body.

In fact, symptoms can worsen before they improve. After diet change, the body's elimination systems have strengthened and gained greater ability to discharge. The extra discharge can cause symptoms to temporarily worsen. These phases of healing are the most difficult. It is discouraging to radically change one's diet and then experience worsening symptoms. During this phase of my healing, my condition was more painful and itched more than I had ever experienced. Four months into diet change, night itching was so terrible that I often wanted to jump out of my skin. I understood how un-resolved itch could drive someone insane. My ankles were so tight and hot that I had to sleep with my feet off the edge of the bed. The heat and the itching regu-larly woke me up in the middle of the night. This was un-doubtedly the most challenging phase of my healing. I had given up so many beloved foods and the social experiences that went along with them, only to see my condition worsening. To stay focused, I read and reread pages in books on natural healing that explained that this type of flare up was an indication that I was healing and releasing more discharge from within. I persisted and after six weeks my healing took a huge turn for the better. Symptoms began to vanish and I have remained in remission for years.

Once your symptoms clear and you experience the incredible healing power of food, you'll be aware of a multitude of potential benefits:

1) The emotional relief that comes from having control over your health and symptoms. This might be the first time you've experienced any control over your symptoms and the disease.

2) You'll be less dependent upon prescription medications and liberated from a very complicated medical system.

3) You'll have more money in your pocket. Your food costs will probably decrease when you buy less meat, dairy and alcohol. Fewer prescription medications and fewer trips to the doctor inevitably mean more money in your pocket, too.

4) If you have other health problems, they might improve, too. For instance, I had chronic allergy problems and sinus infections before changing my diet. A lifetime of allergy problems are now virtually gone.

5) I always emphasize alleviating the cause of disease over weight loss. But you can expect to lose weight and experience the positive health and self-image benefits of weight loss.

But to achieve natural healing with food, I must stress the combined importance of a deliberate diet, patience and persistence. All three are equally critical for success.

Chapter 4
Healing Principles – Diet, Positive Outlook, Activity

"Man must cease attributing his problems to his environment, and learn again to exercise his will—his personal responsibility." Albert Einstein

Many healing diets offer a multipronged approach to true health. Almost all iterate the importance of being in harmony within your own body and within the larger forces of nature. In addition to diet they emphasize the significance of a positive outlook, a grateful attitude and symbiotic interaction with nature. In theory they might say that according to each individual, no food is prohibited and no food alone will heal. However, my humble opinion is that they often reflect an extreme position which strictly forbids many foods and practices. Perhaps because of their demands across every dimension of life, I wasn't surprised at the frequency with which I heard reports of binging and abandonment of these diets. And I've heard a growing list of stories on how strict dietary adherence has been connected to making some people sick.

My intent is to help you bridge the distance between these extremes and what you can realistically accomplish. You should feel good about your achievement—even when it's not perfect. After an initial six month period of cleansing, I encourage flexibility because flexibility is crucial for long-term compliance. And long-term compliance is necessary for natural healing because the process is inherently slow. My hunch is that this orientation will minimize binging and facilitate a more positive outlook, which in turn will enhance the chances of accepting this way of eating for the rest of your life. *For it's what we choose to eat on a daily basis over many years that is the key to preventing and reversing disease naturally with food.*

The tenets of how to eat for good health are neither trendy nor new. They're the same dietary recommendations that we've already heard a million times before, namely:

1) Increase consumption of complex carbohydrates (especially whole grains and fresh vegetables and fresh fruits) and reduce consumption of refined sugars (white sugar, cane juices, high fructose corn syrups, etc);

2) <u>Decrease consumption of animal foods like meats, poultry, eggs and dairy</u>;

3) <u>Reduce total fat consumption, especially of saturated fats</u> which are found in animal products like meat, poultry, eggs and dairy;

4) Eat from a <u>wide variety</u> of <u>fresh foods</u> to secure a balance of vitamins and minerals, thereby decreasing or eliminating the need for supplementation;

5) Eat more <u>high fiber, simple, fresh and organic foods</u> and less chemically processed foods.

Other Healing Principles:

Simplicity:

Throughout history, religious and philosophical leaders have emphasized the value of simplicity. Simple food in its fresh, whole form contains more nutrition than the same food item after it has been processed. Before the advent of pesticides, genetic modifications, grain feed for livestock, artificial colors and flavors and sweeteners, supplemental hormones and antibiotics, bleached flours and such, humans everywhere ate the simple foods designed by nature for consumption. And until the 20th century, everything eaten by humans was organic. We should be mindful of disregarding the wisdom of nature and what we are designed to consume.

Chewing:

Chew your food fifty times or more until it becomes liquid in your mouth. Saliva contains the alkaline enzyme, amylase, which facilitates digestion. The more we chew, the more we release amylase. Chewing also stimulates movement and flow within the lymph nodes under the chin. Some macrobiotic teachers have said that chewing your food more than fifty times can cut healing time in half.

Moderation and Avoidance of Extremes:

Be prepared for hunger. In other words, always keep quality snacks at your fingertips. I overeat and make my worst choices when I'm hungry and not prepared for it. Eat when you're hungry but try to avoid eating three hours before sleeping in order to give your digestive system a break. Avoid overeating. The notion of balance relies on universal harmony and balance instead of extremes in foods, thought and environment. Do the diet imperfectly, without beating yourself up, so that you can do it longer. I believe that the key to healing with food is the ability to persist, so maintain one or two 'sacred' foods to avoid constant feelings of deprivation. For example, I continue to drink coffee every morning as a way to trick my brain into feeling indulged instead of deprived. I believe we're much more prone to binging and abandoning diets when we feel constantly deprived and restricted, so it's important to circumvent those negative emotions with some flexibility.

Food Preparation:

From the standpoint that you are what you eat, we absorb nutrition and vibration from our foods. Consider the inevitable impact of highly refined and processed foods that are designed to maximize profit instead of nutrition. Consider the stable or chaotic energy sources you're using to heat your food, and how that energy transmits into your life. Returning to a simpler way of eating that respects the life-giving quality of food is essential to recovering and maintaining good health and high spirits.

Positive Outlook:

It's no surprise that approaching diet change in an optimistic way will make it easier to accept and practice. However, adopting this diet was the most difficult thing I have ever done. Patience, persistence and right thinking are critical to sustain successful diet change. This lifestyle change may be one of the most demanding changes of your life because food serves to provide not only nutrition, but comfort, pleasure and social context. To radically alter how one eats requires not only a change in food but also a change in attitude that respects one's body and expects true health and happiness to follow self-discipline.

Progress is rarely linear so I constantly remind my clients that this process is "two steps forward, one step back". To stay focused despite inevitable setbacks and occasional binges, it's important to habitually give yourself affirmative messages. When I craved wine, sweets, and spicy foods, I'd repeat positive messages like, "I choose to eat for health. Every day I'm getting better and the diet is easy to follow." Instead of beating yourself up for temporary binges, focus on the positives and regularly congratulate yourself on your examples of self-discipline.

Good, Better Best:
This principle represents the decision process we have in food selection. I love this principle because it refrains from labeling "bad" decisions and instead focuses on positives that leave no associated guilt. Depending upon our commitment level at the moment we choose to eat, we make "good, better, or best" choices.

Chapter 5
Why a Healing Diet Works and the Acid Alkaline Balance

"The human body functions best when our blood is slightly alkaline. We make acid as a natural by-product of metabolism, but we make no alkaline. We must therefore get alkalinizing minerals from our diets."—<u>Cancer Battle Plan Sourcebook</u>, *Dr.* Dave Frahm, 2000, Penguin Putnam Inc., New York, page 147.

"Any stressor that the mind or body interprets and internalizes as too much to deal with, leaves an acid residue. Even a mild stressor can cause a partial or total acid-forming reaction," <u>Alkalize or Die</u>, Dr. Theodore A. Baroody, Jr., 1993, Eclectic Press, Waynesville, NC 28786, page 157.

We've talked about how removing irritating foods and pollutants from the diet will allow intestines to heal and stop more toxins from seeping into the bloodstream. The consumption of certain foods and a positive outlook provide the necessary fiber, nutrition and environment to allow the body to heal and ward off future disease. If toxins continue to be ingested, intestines continue to leak these poisons into the bloodstream creating hyperacidity and a potentially damaging pH in the body. On a scale of zero to fourteen, pH is simply a measurement of alkalinity or acidity and seven is considered neutral. A pH above seven is alkaline and a pH below 7 is acidic.

With pH effects in mind, a balanced healthy lifestyle supports proper alkalinity via consciousness in diet, thought and activity. A healing diet is based around mineral rich plant foods and mineral waters that promote alkalinity. A positive outlook creates positive emotions and the ability to visualize the desired result. Habitually negative, damaging thoughts influence our internal biochemistry and produce acidic toxins. Activity, especially walking in nature, eases the mind and stimulates circulatory, respiratory and lymphatic systems. Laughter and exercise expel carbon dioxide which is mildly acidic. **Diet, thought and exercise are all vital to creating the necessary alkaline internal environment for natural healing.**

First, a healing diet strongly emphasizes mineral rich foods that support proper alkalinity in the body. The majority of one's food intake should consist of alkaline-forming foods, namely organic vegetables and fruits. Chapter Six provides great detail on these alkaline-forming foods, how to find them, and how to integrate them into your lifestyle. Most vegetables, fruits, herbs and sprouts are alkaline-forming, as are almonds and some whole grains. By calling them "alkaline-forming", this means that they render an alkaline ash. By ash, I mean that the remains of digestion are an ash, just like the remains of a burned log on a fire are an ash. That ash has an acidic or an alkaline pH.

Heavier, fattier foods like meat, dairy, fish, and eggs, along with processed foods, grains, refined sugars and refined flours yield an acidic ash. A diet that's high in acid-forming foods, combined with destructive emotions and inactivity, render an overly acidic and disease-prone condition. A plant based diet of mineral rich foods, along with a positive outlook and regular physical activity will support alkalinity, a strong immune system and optimal health. In general, alkaline-forming foods are strongly preferred, but inclusion of some acid-forming foods in the diet is essential for complete nutrition. When you are trying to recover naturally from disease, it is good to have a diet that is roughly 80% alkaline-forming and 20% acid-forming. This will enhance the ability of your immune system to rid your body of toxins and create natural healing. After symptoms are resolved, you still want a majority of your intake to be alkaline-forming. A general guideline for maintaining optimal health is a diet of 60% alkaline-forming and 40% acid-forming foods.

On a separate but important note, when one's diet is acid-forming, the body inevitably has to deplete minerals from other sources to neutralize the excess acid. Bone calcium represents the body's largest and most readily available storage of alkalizing minerals. Calorie for calorie, most dark, leafy green vegetables deliver more calcium than milk. Additionally, the saturated fat and high protein content in dairy contributes directly to acidity. After a little research you'll find that societies which drink milk regularly suffer a higher incidence of osteoporosis than those with dairy-free diets. When people ask me how they'll get enough calcium in their diet if they stop eating dairy products, I ask them to consider how a cow gets all the calcium it needs to make all of those dairy products. Cows don't eat dairy. They are supposed to eat grass, otherwise known as a dark, leafy green vegetable.

Chapter 6
Diet Basics

"Nothing will benefit human health and increase the chances for survival on Earth as much as the evolution to a vegetarian diet."
Albert Einstein

DIET BASICS

- I am neither vegetarian nor vegan. I occasionally eat meat, eggs, fish and dairy. But my diet is overwhelmingly characterized by plant-based foods including whole grains, fresh vegetables and fresh fruits, beans, lentils, seeds and nuts. When in doubt, eat an unprocessed plant. Prioritize a plant-based diet over an organic diet.

- Although I achieved significant healing while buying non-organic produce, subsequent research convinced me of the value of avoiding their genetic modifications, herbicides and pesticides. Now I buy and eat organic produce whenever possible.

- If you suffer from inflammatory diseases like psoriasis, eczema, asthma, allergies, and arthritis, you may want to avoid nightshades and citrus fruits for a few months to observe your response to them. Nightshades include all tomatoes, white potatoes, tobacco, eggplant, and any variety of peppers including bell, jalapeno, serrano, poblano, habanero, etc. Black pepper is not a nightshade. Solanine in nightshades appears to contribute to the inflammatory response in some people. Citrus fruits include oranges, grapefruits, pineapple, lemons and lime.

- Avoid shellfish and filter-feeding fish (like shrimp, lobster, scallops, oysters, clams) as they feed off the sewage that floats down to them. Pollution in our waters has contributed to toxic levels of mercury and other metals in the entire wild fish supply, too. Consumption of freely swimming fish should be limited to eight ounces per week.

- Simple foods and shorter ingredient labels are better. Once a food is no longer in its whole state, it has to be processed in some way to keep it from deteriorating. Fresh is always best, and frozen is the next best option. Canned, dried and fried foods should be rarely eaten.

- Drink filtered, mineral or spring water instead of chlorinated tap water. The chlorine in tap water kills the good bacteria in our gut. Additionally, tap water frequently contains toxic residues, pharmaceuticals and metals.

- Ponder the word 'intoxicated'. As a highly toxic substance, alcohol can kill much faster than terminal diseases like cancer. Especially while attempting to recover from active disease, avoid all alcohol including wine, beer and liquor.

- Avoid products made with refined white sugars, high fructose corn syrup and limit any type of cane juice.

- Check with your physician before embarking upon significant diet change.

- If you determine you are allergic to a food, avoid it even if it is on this list. Many people have intolerances to gluten, corn, soy, shellfish, nuts and casein. Those with gluten intolerance should avoid all wheat, barley, oats, rye, spelt and kamut. "Gluten –free" oats are not considered a risk-free food for those most sensitive to gluten.

- It is my opinion that whole food from nature offers superior nutrition to supplements which have been isolated in a laboratory. We are designed to eat food. There is no substitute for a good diet.

- READ INGREDIENT LABELS LIKE A HAWK! Tricky marketing exists in many areas of "healthy" food products. Simple foods and shorter ingredient labels are better. Choose products made of recognizable foods instead of synthetic laboratory ingredients with unfamiliar names.

- Don't let yourself get hungry. When I'm really hungry and don't have quality food at my fingertips, I invariably get frustrated and overeat whatever is available. Pack healthy snacks in your refrigerator, car, purse and office to ensure you always have quality food at your fingertips. Almond butter, raisins, bars made of whole foods, smoothies made of pureed fruit, and brown rice cakes are great snacks which can travel almost anywhere.

- I always encourage a plant-based diet of simple, whole foods to prevent disease and promote more natural healing. Neverthe-less, personal preference and professional experience highlights that most of us are fundamentally unwilling to permanently exclude all animal products such as beef, chicken, fish, fowl, game, dairy, butterfat and eggs. Rare or occasional consumption of animal products is sensible and appropriate within the context of a healing diet. Indeed some people may or will need more animal product than others and individual needs can change over time. When possible, opt to eat animal products as humans have eaten them throughout human history. In other words, opt for wild ocean fish in lieu of farm raised fish. Opt for grass-fed beef and wild game, or organic meats and dairy and eggs which are free of hormones, antibiotics and genetically modified feed. Consider how the impact of a child's environment impacts his or her future health and why that would ap-ply for the animals that we eat, too. If craved, try to limit yourself to four ounces per week of red meat, eight ounces per week of white chicken or fowl, and two eggs per week.

- Sometimes recovery requires strict removal of dietary casein, a protein found in mam-malian milk and milk products. In this in-

stance I recommend 100% removal of all casein from the diet. Ghee is not considered a
risk-free food for those who need to remove
all casein from their diet. When dietary casein poses no problem I recommend limit-
ing oneself to eight ounces of low- or nonfat
organic yogurt and two ounces of organic or
European cheeses per week.

**Rough dietary guidelines include approximately
25% of daily calories in whole grains; 20% in vegetables; 20% in seeds or nuts or beans or fish; 20%
in fruit; and 15% in oils.**

Whole Grains:
Whole grains comprise approximately 25% of
daily food intake. Except in cases of gluten intolerance,
any whole grains are allowed and brown rice acts as
the daily whole grain staple. Whole grain varieties include brown rice, corn, millet, amaranth, kamut, teff,
spelt, oatmeal, buckwheat, kasha, bulgar, quinoa, triti-
cale, wheat, barley, rye.

From a nutritional standpoint, whole grains are
best and less processing is always better. Each step
of processing or refining a food will devitalize it and
compromise its nutrition. Hence, brown rice is superior
to brown rice flour, steel cut oats are superior to oatmeal flakes, fresh corn is superior to corn meal. White

flour and other highly refined and polished grains are always avoided. Whole grain flours are acceptable on an occasional basis in bagels, breads, muffins, cereals. Gluten intolerance appears to be an issue in several autoimmune diseases like psoriasis. I emphasize brown rice and quinoa as my primary grains.

Vegetables:

About 20% of the daily food should include vegetables and sea vegetables. Vegetables can be prepared in any number of ways including soups, but frying should be avoided. Opinions differ on whether it's better to eat raw versus lightly cooked vegetables, but overcooking vegetables will definitely compromise their nutrition. I try to eat most of my vegetables raw.

All vegetables are allowed. Dark, leafy green vegetables are to be eaten as often as possible as they are very alkalizing. These dark, leafy vegetables include bok choy, arugula, kale, turnip greens, mustard greens, collard greens, watercress, herbs like basil and parsley and cilantro, leeks, spinach, lettuce varieties, chinese cabbage, carrot tops, daikon tops, beet tops, swiss chard, scallions, dandelion greens, broccoli rabe, pak choy and chinese gai lan. Other allowable vegetables include sweet potatoes, yams, string and wax beans, endive, escarole, red and green cabbage, mushrooms, artichokes, carrots, onions, garlic, shallots, sugar snap peas, broccoli, cauliflower, brussel sprouts, asparagus, parsnips, turnips, corn, all squashes, zucchini, beets, olives, celery, fennel, cucumber, garlic, and avocado.

Vegetable soups can be made from any vegetables. (It is ideal to season the soup with miso, but never add miso to boiling water because boiling water will kill the good bacteria in it.) Vegetable soups, bean soups and grain soups are all recommended.

Sea vegetables are frequently used in sushi, miso soup or when cooking rice. Nori, wakame, kombu, hijiki, arame, dulse, kelp, sea palm and Irish moss are all sea vegetables. These veggies are dense with minerals and therefore very alkalizing. Try to include at least a small portion of these in your daily diet. I've not developed a taste for them so I'm always looking for ways to eat them without tasting them. For instance, I'll cook brown rice with kombu, shake dulse granules onto salads and rice dishes, snack on brown rice cakes with seaweed, and dip nori sheets into hummus. Sea vegetables are essentially dark, leafy green vegetables which have derived their mineral density from the ocean floor and seawater. They are alkalizing superfoods. Add them in any way possible to your daily diet.

Seeds, Nuts, Beans and Fish:
For quality protein, about 20% of daily food includes any variety of lentils, seeds, nuts and beans. Wild

fish, wild game, organic meats and eggs can be included on a limited basis. Almonds are considered by some to be the only alkalizing nuts but I eat a wide variety of nuts regularly. Organic tofu, tempeh, seitan and natto, all of which are soybean products, may be taken regularly but in small amounts given estrogenic properties. Grilled, baked, sauteed, steamed or poached wild fish and wild game or organic poultry are recommended at up to six ounces per week. Organic eggs are limited to two eggs per week. Research indicates that large fish including swordfish and salmon can be high in toxic mercury. I avoid the largest fish like swordfish entirely. Now I rarely eat fish. In the beginning I ate light chunk tuna or wild salmon at a maximum of six ounces per week.

Fruit:

About 20% of daily intake comes from fruits, and whole fruit is always preferable to juices because whole fruit provides beneficial fiber and minerals. Nevertheless, if you drink juice, make sure that it's fresh and includes no refined sugars or cane juice.

All fruits are allowed. Fruits that are frozen and packed in water or fruit juice are permitted on occasion but fresh is always best. Strawberries and citrus fruits (oranges, orange juice, grapefruits, pineapple, lemon and limes) are often discouraged for arthritis, psoriasis and psoriatic arthritis. Freshly squeezed lemon or lime can be added to drinking water or used in dressings for a cleansing and alkalizing effect.

Oils:

Quality fat and oils comprise approximately 15% of daily caloric intake. Olive oil is my favorite oil. I adore avocado and my diet includes a fair bit of fat from whole and blended nuts or seeds. Occasionally I consume sesame or peanut oil and occasionally I eat meat or quality cheeses. Salad dressings are best with olive oil and fresh squeezed lemon juice or raw apple cider vinegar. If possible and if the recipe allows it, I cook without oil and then add olive oil after a food is cooked. Macadamia nut and coconut oils are known for their ability to sustain nutrition integrity at higher temperatures.

Note:

Registered dietitians including Jenna Wunder, MPH, RD, and medical doctors at the University of Michigan's Integrative Medicine Department have developed a **"Healing Foods Pyramid"** with very similar guidelines. Please visit their user-friendly website at www.med.umich.edu/umim for helpful suggestions and detailed information.

Always Limit or Avoid:

Non-organic beef and non-organic chicken and their fats. Non-organic dairy and dairy milk fat. All white sugar, corn syrups and cane juices. All white flour. More than one glass of wine per week. More than one cup of coffee per day. Nitrates, nitrites and all processed meats like bacon, bologna, sausage and hot dogs. Tobacco. Shellfish like shrimp, lobster, oysters and scallops which are filter feeders that consume sewage from the sea floor. Junk food and processed foods like sodas. Trans-fatty acids and partially hydrogenated fats in packaged foods and fast foods. All fried foods. Sweets and pastries. Artificial sweeteners like Splenda and Aspartame. Artificial colors and MSG preservatives. Sugary cereals made with sugar and cane juice. Extremely spicy foods.

Chapter 7
Grocery Shopping

Shopping can be overwhelming when you revise your dietary choices to minimize or eliminate dairy, chicken, red meat, wheat, sodas, alcohol, nightshades, sweets, and refined flour products. In an attempt to make shopping easier for you, this chapter provides lists of foods and their general location. This list is by no means representative of the only things I buy. This list provides general guidelines to help you understand how to make grocery store choices anywhere.

General shopping suggestions include:

1) If particular foods are especially tempting because they're associated with your old habits or addictions, avoid them altogether. Don't even look at them. I try to completely avoid the bakery section and sheet cakes because that thick, butter cream icing is my biggest temptation.

2) Don't go to the grocery store hungry. Even if you don't feel hungry before going to the store, eat something in advance of shopping to lessen impulsive temptations.

3) Buy some items that aren't exactly perfect to allow for occasional moments of feeling indulged rather than deprived.

4) Keep a few prized items on hand at all times to decrease your chances of binging. For example, in the past, I didn't allow myself the expense of precut fresh fruit. Then I realized that by eliminating animal products and alcohol, I save more than enough money to buy precut fruits. Keeping some precut fruit in my refrigerator ensures that I always have something sweet and nutritious at my fingertips for those times when I'm craving sweetness. I also buy bars with ingredients that are whole and not isolated in a laboratory. Their ingredients usually include nuts and dried fruits, and they travel well. If I'm on a road trip or stuck in traffic, or at a party where there's nothing good to eat, or I'm nowhere near a grocery store, it's a huge relief to have these bars at my fingertips. Every day seems to include moments when it's impossible to quickly access quality food, so ensure that you're prepared with quality snacks. As my hunger rises, my willpower falls. The key is to be prepared and to avoid feeling starved.

Produce

Organic Spring Mix, Organic Baby Spinach, Organic Carrots and Organic Baby Carrots, Celery, Carrots, Cabbages, Broccoli, Romaine, Sugar Snap Peas, Haricot Verts and Green Beans, Asparagus, Corn, Butternut and Acorn Squash, Zucchini, Summer Squash, Bell Peppers, Brussel Sprouts, Cucumber, Avocado, Onion varieties, Garlic, Sweet Potatoes, Red Potatoes, White Potatoes, Tomato varieties.

Organic Apple varieties, Watermelon, Strawberries, Blackberries, Blueberries, Cherry varieties, Pear varieties, Avocado, Olive varieties, Mango, Pineapple, Bananas, Orange varieties, Lemons, Limes, Plums, Nectarines, Peaches, Dates, Cantaloupe, Precut fruit varieties.

Organic Carrot Juice, Acai Juice, Pomegranate Juice, Fresh squeezed Orange and Grapefruit Juices

Seafood, Meats and Prepared Foods

Fresh Wild Fish Varieties, Smoked Salmon, Ceviche, Organic Ground Beef, Organic Chicken Breasts, Hormone-free Rotisserie Chicken, Braseola, Pickled Herring, Garbanzo Bean Salad, Organic Tofu, Basil Pesto, Organic Hummus, Fresh Salsa Varities, Olive Tapenades, Olive Varieties, Tzatziki, Dolmas

Grocery

Walnuts, Almonds, Peanuts, Pine and Macadamia Nuts, Mixed Nuts, Cashews, Pistachios

Coconut Cashews
Trail Mix Varieties
Olive Varieties
Sardines in Olive Oil
Almond Butter, Organic Peanut Butter, Cashew Butter,
Sun Butter
Gluten free Brown Rice Cake varieties
Honey
100% Organic Maple Syrup
100% Fruit Spread
Organic Brown Rice varieties
Organic Flax Seeds
Dried Cherries, Dried Blueberries, Dried Cranberries,
Dried Berry Mixes
Organic Raisins
Organic Olive Oil
Balsalmic Vinegar
Sun Dried Tomatoes
Marinated Artichokes
Four Bean Salad
Organic Pasta Sauce
Gluten free Pasta
Gluten free Hot Cereals
Organic Apple Sauce
Sea Salt
Japanese Green Tea
Organic Soy, Rice, Almond, Hemp, or Hazelnut Milks
San Pelegrino Mineral Water
100% Fruit Juices

Organic Coffee

European or Organic Cheeses
Goat Cheese Varities
Parmesan Cheese and other hard cheeses

Prepared Snacks
Organic Fruit Roll Ups
Vegetable Chips and Gluten Free Chip varieties
Multigrain Chip varieties
Bars made with whole foods including nuts, seeds, fruit
Trail Mix Varieties
Coconut Cashews
Organic Applesauce

Frozen and Refrigerated Foods
Organic Blackberries, Organic Blueberries, Frozen Strawberry and Berry blends
Organic Blackberry Sorbet
Fruit Sorbets
Frozen Organic Gluten free Meals
Frozen Organic Gluten free Buckwheat Waffles
Wild Fish Varieties
Smoothie Packs
Organic Frozen Vegetable Varieties
Organic Eggs
Greek and organic Yogurt Varieties
Coconut, Rice or Organic Soy Yogurt varieties

Organic Carrot and Vegetable Juices
Pomegranate Juice
Acai Juice

The Dirty Dozen are the twelve most contaminated fruits and vegetables. It's more important to buy organic when buying this specific type of produce. Notice that many on this list are thin skinned.

Apples
Bell peppers
Celery
Cherries
Imported grapes
Nectarines
Peaches
Pears
Potatoes
Red raspberries
Spinach
Strawberries

The 12 Least Tainted fruits and vegetables have a thicker skin and are often eaten peeled. It's less important to buy organic when buying this produce.

Asparagus
Avocados
Bananas

Broccoli
Cauliflower
Sweet corn
Kiwi
Mangos
Onions
Papaya
Pineapples
Sweet peas

Chapter 8
In My Refrigerator

Precut fruit varieties
Strawberries, Blackberries or Blueberries
Watermelon
Lemons
Apple Varieties
Organic Carrot Juice
Acai Juice
Organic Spring Salad Mix, Organic Baby Spinach, Organic Arugula
Organic Baby Carrots
Broccoli Florets
Nondairy beverages like Rice, Almond or Hemp Milks
Organic Hummus
Dolma
Organic Eggs
100% Maple Syrup
Olive Varieties
Pesto Varieties
Sundried Tomatoes
Organic Applesauce
Precut Vegetables
Organic Sesame Oil
French Mustard

Organic Miso
Organic Tofu
Italian Parmesian Cheese
Greek Feta Cheese
San Pelegrino Mineral Water
Marinated Artichokes
Four Bean Salad
Organic Eggs
Pickled Herring
Organic Peanut Butter
Almond Butter, Sunflower Seed Butter, Organic Peanut Butter

Other Produce: Celery, Shallots, Onions, Chives, Garlic, Beets, Leeks, Turnips, Avocado, Romaine, Limes, Lemons, Squash Varieties, Haricot Verts and Green Beans, Corn, Rapini, Sugar Snap Peas, Asparagus, Burdock Root, Daikon, Kale Varieties, Sweet Potatoes, Yams, Fennel.

In My Freezer:
Frozen Organic Blackberries and Berry Mixes
Organic Coffee
Frozen Organic Blackberry Sorbet Bars

In My Pantry:
Pinto Beans
Brown Rice Cake Varieties
Locally produced Honey

Sardines in Lemon Juice and Olive Oil
Nut and Seed Varieties
Dried Fruit Varieties
Black pepper, Sea Salt and Tumeric
Snack Bars made with nuts, seeds, dried fruits, raw
chocolate
Green Tea
Organic, Cold Pressed Olive Oil
Balsalmic Vinegar
Himalayan Sea Salt
Rice or Corn Crackers and Chips
Gluten-Free Pastas
Rice Noodles
Organic Dry Popped Popcorn

Chapter 9
In Austin Restaurants

An increasing number of restaurants offer meals of brown rice, fresh and sautéed vegetables, sea vegetables, vegetable or miso soups, beans and rice, fresh fruit and 100% fruit smoothies, sushi rolls wrapped in nori, gluten-free pastas, grilled ocean fish, grilled fish tacos, mixed greens and salads, rice noodles with tofu and vegetables, grilled fish salads, vegetarian fajitas and nachos, bean dishes and hummus, all natural meats, wild game and fowl. Nevertheless, we don't live in a perfect world where fresh, organic plant-based meals are always at our fingertips. Instead of surrendering in frustration, we can learn the basic guidelines for better meal choices and make them in any restaurant anywhere.

Below is a list of restaurants in Austin, but the general decision principles could be applied in any restaurant anywhere. This list emphasizes restaurants where you can maintain a plant-based diet built around whole grains, vegetables, fruits, beans, lentils, nuts and seeds. If you don't see these things on the menu, ask if they can be made for you. Sometimes restaurants will serve gluten-free and dairy-free items which aren't listed on their menu. Many times I've marveled at the effort restaurant staff will make to meet dietary restrictions. If I encounter any resistance, I use "food allergies" as my excuse for special requests.

- **Zen**—Japanese fast food, brown rice dishes with a wide variety of vegetables

- **Berryhill Baja**—Spinach and corn tamales, rice, beans, guacamole, grilled fish tacos

- **Casa de Luz**—Macrobiotic restaurant and products

- **PeiWei Asian Diner**—Gluten-free and dairy-free options, brown rice

- **Fire Bowl Café**—Brown rice and vegetables

- **East Side Café**—Lots of vegetable side dishes and vegetarian entrees

- **Maria's Taco Xpress**—Vegetarian or bean taco on corn tortilla, guacamole

- **Hyde Park Bar & Grill**—Veggie platter, roasted carrots

- **Madras Pavilion, Swad and All Indian Restaurants**—Vegan options, lentils, rice

- **Guero's Mexican Food**—Corn tortillas, rice, beans, grilled fish and veggies, guacamole

- **Uchi, Benihana and All Japanese Restaurants**

- **Polvo's Mexican Food**—Grilled fish with black beans and rice, guacamole

- **Magnolia Café**—Love Veggies, Black Bean Entrée, grilled fish with brown rice

- **Kerby Lane Café**—All natural beef and chicken, several vegetarian options

- **Wild Woods Gluten-free Café**

- **Luby's**—Baked white fish, salads, veggie side dishes

- **Veggie Heaven**—Brown rice, lots of vegetarian entrees

- **Castle Hill Food for Fitness Cafe**—Healthy food to go

- **Galaxy Café**—Several vegetarian options, fun décor

- **Cosmic Café**—Vegetarian restaurant with Indian spices, formerly the West Lynn Café

- **Ranch 616**—Vegetable Tower, grilled fish with vegetables, customization by request

- **Roy's**—Fabulous grilled fish plates with delicious vegetable side dishes

- **Eddie V's**—Incredible grilled fish plates with delicious vegetable side dishes

- **Souper Salad**—Giant salad bar

- **Fresh Choice**—Giant salad bar

- **Daily Juice and Daily Juice Cafe, Beets Living Foods Cafe**—Raw juices and raw menu options

- **Baby Greens**—Drive through with variety of prepared salads

- **Café Mundi**—Delicious vegetarian entrees and soups, east Austin vibe

- **Bouldin Creek Coffeehouse, Somnio's Cafe**—Vegetarian and gluten-free options with a south Austin vibe

- **Mother's Café and Garden**—Vegetarian restaurant

- **Wahoo's Fish Tacos**—Fish tacos, beans, corn tortillas, pico de gallo, cilantro, avocado

- **Baja Fresh**—Fish tacos, beans, rice, corn tortillas, pico de gallo, cilantro, avocado

- **Mr. Natural**—Wholesome and tasty baked goods, juices, tamales, lunch specials

- **African and Ethiopian Restaurants**—Lentils, rice, beans, greens

- **Alborz, Phoenicia Bakery, Middle Eastern and Greek restaurants**—Persian rice, grilled veggies and lean meats, hummus, baba ganoush, bean salads, falafel

- **Madame Mam's, Thai Noodle, Thai Passion, Thai-Fresh and all Thai restaurants**

- **Sunflower and all Vietnamese Restaurants**—Rice bowls and vegetables

- **Java Noodle and all Indonesian Restaurants**—Rice dishes with vegetables

- **Din Ho and All Chinese Restaurants**—Rice and rice noodles with sautéed vegetables

- **Italian Restaurants**—Grilled fish & veggies, corn polenta, olives, rice risotto

- **Jamba Juice**—100% fruit smoothies

- **Chipolte**—Burrito Bowl with black beans, rice, guacamole and lemon squeezed on top

- **Chango's**—Grilled mahi mahi tacos on corn tortillas with black beans

- **Freebird**—Bird Salad or tacos with black beans and rice on corn tortillas

- **Boston Market**—Numerous vegetable side dishes, fruit cup, salads, soups

- **California Pizza Kitchen**—Creative salads and soups

- **Taco Cabana**—Rice, black beans, cilantro, pico de gallo

- **Outback Steakhouse**—Baked sweet potato, vegetable side dishes, salads, grilled fish

- **Panera**—Salads, soups

- **Oaxacan Tamaleo**—Corn tamales with black beans wrapped in a banana lead

- **Dandelion Cafe**—Black bean chalupas, beans and brown rice, Mediterranean plate

- **Austin Java Co.**—Wonderful salads, smoothies, omelettes, coffees

- **Noodlism**—Lots of rice and vegetable options

- **Mandola's Italian Market**—Yummy prepared bean and vegetable salads to go

Chapter 10
On a Trip

For traveling, you can pack:

Brown rice cakes, almond butter, local honey, fresh fruit, fresh fruit spreads, fruit juice sweetened cereal, almond milk, hummus, canned tuna, precut veggie sticks, snack bars, vegetarian sushi (with no perishable meat or fish in it), brown rice and precut veggie mixes, salad dressing of vinegar and oil, seeds (pumpkin, sunflower), nuts (almonds, pistachios, walnuts, pecans), raisins, dried fruits, wheat-free fig bars, chips and popcorn.

Pack a cooler with:
1) Ice
2) Nondairy beverages like almond milk – individual portions are best but these might only be available in soy milk. With soy milk, it's harder to find options that don't include cane juice. If you are very serious about healing, get rice or almond milk without cane juice. Keep the rice or almond milk in the cooler with ice. If you use individual portions, you don't have to keep them refrigerated until they're opened.

3) Lemons and Olive Oil for salad dressing
4) Cooked brown rice in a Tupperware container. Just add precut veggies and dressing to this to make a delicious and quick meal.
5) Precut, prepackaged veggies – pack these on top of a cooler so they don't get wet, and take some freezer bags or Tupperware containers to keep the melted ice out. You can dip these in almond butter or hummus and add them to rice dishes or eat them plain.
6) Prepackaged salad greens – add as many dark, leafy veggies as possible. Make a salad or add them on top of dishes.
7) Individual portion 100% fruit juices
8) If you can really keep things cold, you may want to take nonfat or coconut yogurt.
9) Fresh fruit that you prefer to eat cold, like grapes.

If you can't have a cooler, all of this will probably hold a few days in a refrigerated hotel room that's shaded from direct sunlight. Put the products as near to the cold air from the air conditioner as possible. If you take yogurt, the organic ones which contain only nonfat milk and cultures seem to survive best.

Dry packing:
1) Fruit juice sweetened Cereal
2) Canned or vacuum packed Light Tuna

3) Canned Sardines
4) Rice or nonwheat crackers
5) Packaged plain oatmeal
6) Almonds, sliced or whole, to add to hot breakfast cereals
7) Seeds and nuts to add to dishes and to eat as snacks
8) Any dried and unsweetened fruits
9) Snack bars and fig bars
10) Individually portioned fruit juices and fresh fruit
11) Almond butter, 100% fruit spreads and local honey
12) Brown Rice Cakes with Seaweed
13) One plate, fork, spoon, knife and reusable cloth napkin per person.
14) Distilled, spring or mineral water

Chapter 11
What to Expect

1) Your stools should change for the better. You should have at least one to two formed stools per day without straining.

2) Over time, you can expect a weird discharge. As the body increases its ability to eliminate accumulated toxins, they will come out through stools and other areas such as skin, lungs and reproductive organs. This might be evidenced by a different and heavier menstruation, rashes or a brownish discharge from the skin, or flu-like symptoms. Discharges are temporary but you'll notice them because they will be unusual.

3) When embarking upon a major lifestyle change, it is imperative to surround yourself with supportive people who will facilitate, rather than complicate, your natural healing. Eliminating or minimizing alcohol and animal products from one's diet can present challenges of social acceptance from family and friends. Tell them about your decision to

use food in pursuit of more natural healing. Ask for their help and give them specific suggestions on how they can support you and increase your chances of success. For example, suggest specific restaurants, let friends know you'll bring a dish to dinner parties that everybody can try, perhaps even ask them to refrain from eating things in front of you that present the biggest temptation.

4) In physical and emotional ways, food and dietary habits are like addictions. Understanding and accepting this before you embark upon diet change will make it easier to move past the anger, withdrawal and feelings of deprivation when they arise. Utilize affirmative statements to counteract these negative feelings. Try to focus on the good your body offers you and be grateful for that, rather than focusing on the illness and dietary restrictions you might be facing.

5) Be prepared to get hungry. My worst choices happen when I'm hungry and unprepared for it. Always keep healthy foods at your fingertips and in your car, purse, home and office to avoid instances when hunger hits and it's impossible to go to the grocery store.

Larabars, Cliff Bars, Roasted Peanuts, Brown Rice Cakes and Almond Butter, Almonds and Raisins, and fruit smoothies all work for me.

6) To give natural healing with food a chance to succeed, I believe it's important to have a very high level of commitment to it for at least six months. Attempt to rarely deviate during that timeframe. After six months and after you've experienced symptom improvement, allow yourself more flexibility. For instance, I was extremely compliant and never ate nightshades for the first six months. Now I have nightshades about once a week. I also eat beef and chicken about 4 times per year, sometimes more, and I drink wine about 3 times per year. For long-term success with this diet, I believe it helps to do the diet imperfectly. This will allow you to practice a healing diet longer, and it will also ensure that you get a wide variety of nutrients in your diet. I guard one or two cherished foods, like coffee in the morning, to trick my brain from feelings of deprivation and to make it easier to accept practicing this diet for the rest of my life.

Chapter 12
Recipe-free Meals and Snacks

Breakfast:

1) Whole Grain Cereals. Read ingredient labels to avoid cane juice.
2) Sliced Fresh Fruit
3) Steel Cut Oats – with or without raisins, pumpkin seeds, sunflower seeds, sliced fruit, diced dried fruits like apricots, cherries, cranberries. Including a good protein source like seeds or nuts in the cereal will sustain you for a longer period of time before hunger hits again. Steel cut oats are especially recommended for those with heart disease and elevated cholesterol levels. For those who want to practice a gluten-free diet, oats are not recommended. Gluten-free hot cereals are available in quinoa, brown rice, buckwheat.
4) Breakfast Bar made of only nuts and seeds and dried fruit. Avoid cane juice and processed items which have been isolated in a

laboratory. Wheat-free, fruit sweetened fig bars smeared with organic peanut butter.

5) Rice or Almond Milk – Always look for the labels which do not include any cane juice. These beverages are presented as alternatives to dairy milk because many people have allergies to casein, a protein found in mammalian dairy and dairy products. Dairy is mucus-forming, meaning that it slows down the elimination process versus facilitating it. For many, mammalian dairy products should be limited or avoided. Nondairy beverages include rice, almond, hazelnut, hemp, soy, and coconut "milks".

6) Pureed fruit smoothies and fruit juices. Brown Rice Drinks without cane juice.

7) Breakfast at one of the listed restaurants.

Lunch and Dinner:

1) Cooked brown rice is always in my refrigerator. Put Precut Vegetables (Chinese Veggie Mix, Coleslaw, Broccoli Slaw, etc) atop brown rice (or any cooked whole grain). Add variety by alternating various precut veggies and salad dressings.

2) Take the same dish above except add your own vegetables with or without more precut vegetables. I often cook brown rice

with turnips and sweet potato and yams. To make the rice, I use two parts water to one part brown rice with sea salt and an ice-cube sized chunk of kombu. Bring the rice and water to a boil, turn the temperature down very low to maintain a slow boil, put the lid on the pot and set the timer for approximately thirty five minutes. The rice is done when there's no standing water in the bottom of the pot. When the rice has finished cooking, I turn off the heat, remove the kombu and top the steaming brown rice with chopped vegetables of any kind. (Then I give the cooked kombu to my dog so that he'll get extra minerals, too.) I put the lid back on to cover everything in the pot so that the steam from the rice will lightly cook the rest of the vegetables. My favorite vegetables for this dish are asparagus, fresh cut corn from the husk, carrots, burdock root, daikon radish, celery, bok choy, green cabbage, beets, kale, beets, turnips, collard greens, arugula and scallions. I always put the dark leafy greens at the top of the pot so that they steam the least. Serve on a bed of mixed salad greens or arugula, sprinkle with dulse granules and gomasio, and then top it with your favorite dressing.

3) Hummus wrapped in a corn tortilla with mixed greens and arugula.

4) Miso Soup with wakame.

5) Tuna Salad made with lemon juice and olive oil or vegetarian "mayonnaise" with any mixture of many vegetables. I mix in broccoli slaw, coleslaw, carrots, grapes, seeds, celery, fresh cut corn and tumeric. Then I wrap this tuna salad in a corn tortilla.

6) Brown rice cakes with seaweed, almond butter and 100% fruit spread, fresh fruit, dried fruit or honey.

7) Brown rice cakes with tamari and seaweed, roasted tahini, 100% fruit spread or fresh fruit or honey.

8) For a quick soup, you can use any fresh or frozen vegetable. Place in a pot, cover the veggies with water, add sliced onions and celery and sea salt and pepper, bring to a boil and cook until done. Puree the cooked vegetables for a delicious pureed soup. Garnish with cilantro, scallions or parsley.

9) Sardines in olive oil with rice crackers.

10) Fresh veggie plate with hummus or pesto and olives.

11) Ethiopian Teff bread with mild lentils and spinach side dishes.

12) Steel cut oats or hot quinoa with sunflower seeds or sliced almonds, dried or fresh fruit, flax seeds.

13) Recommended cereal with a banana or another fruit and almond milk.

14) Fruit smoothie with nonfat, organic, plain yogurt, frozen fruit of choice and organic apple juice.

15) Precut fruit and vegetables and organic goat cheese with fresh squeezed lemon juice.

16) Steamed white fish with any assortment of vegetables on a bed of mixed greens.

17) Any of the restaurants provided.

Snacks:

1) Brown Rice Cakes – Tamari with Seaweed is the best choice. They also make fabulous brown rice chips with sesame and seaweed.

2) Almond Butter with 100% fruit spreads on a brown rice cake. 100% fruit is recommended over honey, but honey is a much better choice than a white sugar alternative. You can also add whole fruit, raisins, agave nectar.

3) Any nut butter which includes just the nuts and sea salt (i.e. the fewest ingredients possible). Almonds are the best nut because they are the only nut which yields alkalinity.

4) Breads and tortillas with fewer ingredients. Compare ingredient labels and you'll see the difference. In general, shorter ingredient lists indicate less processing.

5) Various chips made with puffed rice, root vegetables, spinach, kale.

6) Snack bars and granola bars which are sweetened with honey and contain no cane sweeteners. Roasted peanuts in the shell. Tamari roasted almonds and raw or roasted seeds.

7) Coconut date rolls.

8) Steamed organic Edamame with sea salt.

9) Wheat-free, fruit juice sweetened, raspberry fig bars.

10) Corn chips and other brands with a short ingredient list including only corn, corn oil, sea salt. Organic, dry popped popcorn with sea salt.

11) Toasted tamari almonds and raisins.

12) Nori sheets dipped in hummus and home-made sushi with your choice of vegetables and sauces. Sushi is relatively easy to make and would be a fun project for kids.

13) Puffed and fruit sweetened cereal options including Organic Millet, Puffed Corn and Puffed Brown Rice.

14) Vegetable soup with any vegetables. Chop the vegetables, add them to the pot and

cover them with water. It's better to add too little water than too much of it because you can always add more water later. Add sea salt, celery, onions, and garlic. Bring to a boil, cover the pot and simmer on low heat until all vegetables are at your preferred texture. Puree as desired. You can also use frozen vegetables like peas and corn to avoid chopping vegetables. Pasta or rice noodles can be added and it's best to boil the vegetables separately from the noodles. Hard squashes and root vegetables like potatoes and sweet potatoes take longer to cook, so you'll want to throw them in the pot at the beginning. Add miso when desired but be sure to add it AFTER the water has stopped boiling to avoid killing the good bacteria ("probiotics") in it. If you're not accustomed to miso flavor, white miso is sweet and an easier introduction to the flavor of miso than the heavier barley miso. However, the older barley miso offers the best healing benefits.

15) Pureed fruit smoothies and juices without cane juice or refined sugars.

16) Sardines in olive oil on rice crackers.

17) Unsweetened, organic applesauce and apples.

About Deirdre Earls, MBA, RD, LD:

Registered Dietitian Deirdre Earls graduated with Cum Laude honors in Scientific Nutrition and her healthcare career spans nearly thirty years. Having used an imperfect diet instead of chemotherapy to reverse her own disabling disease, now her objective is to use decades of work to help others achieve the healing power of food in the midst of a busy lifestyle. A featured speaker for radio and TV, medical professionals, universities and corporations, Deirdre has been published in Prevention magazine and a documentary of her recovery, "The Incurables", airs nationally on Veria TV. Her private consultations, lectures, books, menu designs, blog and newsletter are designed to help others easily implement a sustainable healing diet anytime and anywhere on the path to remarkable results. For more information please visit www.YourHealingDiet.com or call (512) 453-8784.

Made in the USA
Charleston, SC
12 March 2010